Understanding Hospice and Palliative Care

Copyright © 2012 by Dr. Jerome Cox

ISBN 978-0-9968711-7-4

For orders, bookings, or further information on hospice, please write or call:

St. Mark Hospice & Palliative Care
657 Jordan Street
Shreveport, LA 71101
318-932-1111 or 318-461-7936
jcox@stmarkhospice.com

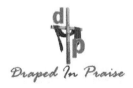

Draped in Praise Publishing & Ministry
PO Box 3231, League City, TX 77573
www.drapedinpraise.org

Dedication

This book is dedicated to my late brother Tony Cox. When you were with us, you had plenty to say as a loving family man, a professional peace officer and a devoted Christian. But it was after you went home that you spoke the loudest.

It was your works – the acts of service you performed for the sick, shut-in, elderly and needy; the thousands of youth to whom you offered loving but firm correction at the most critical times of their lives; and the time, finances and other personal resources which you gave so freely to so many…all without speaking a word about it.

The voice of your heart spoke so loudly to me that I sought to follow your lead, and so began my own campaign of giving. It started with volunteering for hospice; it has culminated in the fulfillment of my dream of owning my own hospice.

I continue to hear your voice every day of my life; my dreams for the future including seeing you face-to-face in the Kingdom; we have so much to talk about!

Introduction

Perhaps more than ever before in our society, we live in a time of never-ending comparisons, contrasts and inequalities. Social media and overall mass communications constantly proclaim and depict the bizarre disproportions of our day. For example, some of our most glamorous cities have department store windows boasting handbags which cost as much as homes. And mere blocks away, there are homeless people sleeping on sidewalks.

Celebrities are regularly compared to each other – as well as to their younger selves as the public mercilessly decides whether they are aging gracefully or not. One 21-year-old is a billionaire pursued by paparazzi; another is buried in college textbooks and living on student loans. One person commits a crime and walks, another commits a seemingly lesser offense and receives a harsh sentence.

Yet, I remain of the opinion that we are all more alike than we are different. Working as a nurse has taught me that when people are ill, injured or dying, they are all the same – human. Their basic needs are the same – healing, relief from pain, and a compassionate person to facilitate those.

We don't need anyone to remind us that death is non-discriminating; everyone will die. This fact alone makes death a topic of premiere importance. However, conversations regarding death are relatively scarce. Even medical professionals receive very little education regarding death, as they are taught primarily to heal.

I have called sickness and death The Great Equalizers; because when they enter the picture, all the qualities that make us different from one another are no longer important...or even relevant. The truth is people who are sick and/or dying are remarkably similar.

Hospice certainly recognizes this – and this recognition allows us to fulfill the third tenet of Hippocrates' famous doctrine concerning what he called the art of medicine – "Cure sometimes, treat often, comfort always."

Linda A. Cox, APRN, FNP-C

Hear My Voice

Table of Contents

Introduction

Chapter 1 – What is Hospice/Palliative Care? 8

Chapter 2 – Your Hospice Team 14

Chapter 3 – What to Expect 18

Chapter 4 – Hospice Myths and Reality 22

Chapter 5 – Stages of Decline and Death 28

Chapter 6 – Comfort You Can Provide........... 36

Chapter 7 – Saying Goodbye 40

Chapter 8 - Hear My Voice ....…..…….. 44

"Suffering is only intolerable when nobody cares…"

\- Cicely Saunders

What are Hospice and Palliative Care?

I am sure that care of the dying has taken place longer than you and I can imagine. Some sources indicate that the concept of hospice goes back as early as the 4th Century AD, when religious institutions welcomed in travelers, as well as the elderly and the ill. History tells us that the word "hospice" came into use in the mid-1800's. Its meaning has Latin and French roots and has to do with the concepts of hospitality and care.

Dame Cicely Mary Saunders was an English doctor, researcher, nurse, social worker, and writer who is known for being the developer of modern hospice and palliative care. In 1963 her famous lecture at Yale University brought discussion of dying and death out into the open. She taught nurses, social workers, chaplains and medical students the importance of addressing "total pain" in terminal patients. This unprecedented concept introduced pain and suffering as being multidimensional in nature. According to Saunders, treating this pain requires holistic care, addressing a patient's physical, sociocultural, emotional and spiritual needs. She placed importance on that care occurring in the patient's home.

Four years later, Saunders founded the world's first modern hospice in the United Kingdom. In 1972, the U.S. Senate

Special Committee on Aging conducted the first national hearing on death with dignity. Testifying at this hearing was Elisabeth Kubler Ross, known today for her Five Stages of Grief.

In the U.S., the first hospice opened in 1974. In 1986 the Medicare Hospice Benefit was created. By the early 1990's, hospice had become an accepted part of healthcare provisions.

At any given time, there are people dying in hospitals and facilities, under circumstances which are inconsistent with their wishes. They may be receiving medications or treatment they do not want. Or, they may have received aggressive therapy for a terminal disease but have continued to decline or suffer pain and other symptoms. Physicians may feel it is time to look at other options such as hospice or palliative care.

Hospice is a philosophy of care that stands unique in the healthcare spectrum. Its focus is on caring rather than curing. People with life-limiting illness can receive holistic care from an interdisciplinary team of professionals who are trained to treat physical pain and provide support for psychosocial, emotional and spiritual needs. This can be accomplished wherever the patient is – at home or in a facility.

To meet patient needs, at all times and in all circumstances, hospice care is provided on four levels:

Routine – This is the most common level of care. In this level, the patient receives routine care in their place of residence.

Continuous – This level of care provides continuous nursing service during a crisis. Nurses, with the help of hospice aides and other caregivers, provide treatment and monitoring for eight to 24 hours daily during a time of acute pain or other symptoms.

Inpatient Respite – This level is designed to care for the patient in a facility, in order to provide a period of relief for the patient's primary caregiver.

General inpatient – This level is utilized when pain and other symptoms cannot be managed in the home. General inpatient care can be provided in a hospital, inpatient hospice facility or in a long-term care facility where nursing personnel are present 24 hours a day.

Regardless of which level, the hospice team delivers expert treatment of pain and other discomforts and provides psychosocial, cultural and emotional/spiritual support for patients and their families. Medications, supplies and equipment needed for this treatment are included in hospice care. These services are available 24 hours a day, seven days a week. After a patient dies, bereavement support is provided for one year.

According to the U.S. Centers for Medicare and Medicaid Services, to qualify for hospice, a patient must be diagnosed with a life-limiting condition, with a life expectancy of six months or less if that illness continues its natural course. Eligibility is verified through hospital records, as well as signs of decline such as frequent hospitalizations, infections, weight loss, increasing weakness, deteriorating mental status and inability to accomplish some or all activities of daily living without assistance.

As stated, hospice services are covered by Medicare, as well as Medicaid in most states. Hospice is also part of the Veterans Administration benefits package. Private insurance generally provides some coverage for hospice care. If the patient has no insurance or benefits, financial assistance is often available through donations, grants, community resources and other sources. All of this will be discussed during the initial hospice consultation.

Palliative Care

Palliative care is specialized care designed to treat pain and discomfort in patients with serious illness. Palliative care provides the same interdisciplinary services as hospice care. But while hospice care begins after aggressive or curative treatments have stopped, patients receiving palliative care can continue their curative treatments while they receive expert management of their pain and other symptoms. Palliative care can begin at any stage of the illness, and eligibility does not depend on prognosis. Care can be given in hospitals, nursing homes and other long-term care facilities, or in the patient's home.

"We are all just walking each other home."

\-   Ram Dass

Your Hospice Team

Hospices are licensed by their state departments of health and accredited through state and national agencies. Hospice care standards have been established by the National Hospice and Palliative Care Organization, and hospices must meet certain Conditions of Participation of the Centers for Medicare Services, in order to receive reimbursements. All hospices undergo regular surveys to ensure compliance with licensing and accreditation standards.

As stated, hospice is a philosophy of care, and services are delivered using an interdisciplinary approach. This means that the physical, psychosocial, emotional/spiritual needs of both patient and family are addressed and cared for by professionals who are specially trained in that discipline.

Hospices are extensively staffed to provide for patient needs. The staff includes an administrator and governing body; a medical director, director of nursing and a host of other professionals including social workers, nurses, counselors and therapists, as well as volunteers. All of these staff members are qualified through education and training specific to their hospice roles. This training is required at the time of hire and is maintained and updated throughout hospice employment.

The hospice caregivers whom you will see most often and on a regular basis, are described as the core team. Your core hospice team is known as the interdisciplinary team, or IDT, and consists of the following:

- **Physician** – A licensed doctor who is responsible for the medical care of the patient. This doctor may be the patient's primary care physician, or the hospice medical director if the PCP has turned over care to him/her. In either case, the hospice medical director works closely with the PCP.

- **Registered nurse** – A licensed RN who is responsible for designing and implementing the patient's personal plan of care. This is accomplished through continuous communication and coordination with other members of the interdisciplinary team (IDT).

- **Social worker** – A licensed social worker with at least a master's degree, who is responsible for assessing the social, economic and psychological/emotional elements related to the patient's health status and needs. Together with other members of the IDT, the hospice social worker endeavors to meet those needs throughout hospice care.

- **Spiritual counselor** – A qualified counselor who is responsible for providing spiritual support, direction and guidance. This counselor is often described as a hospice chaplain; to serve in this role, an individual must possess formal training and skills as evidenced by a Bachelor or Master of Divinity degree, or other theological degree/training from an accredited institution.

- **Volunteer** – Hospice volunteers play a fundamental, very meaningful role in the delivery of hospice care. Volunteers are caring, supportive, non-biased people who assist patients, their families and the hospice program as assigned. Like all other members of the IDT, hospice volunteers are trained and held to the standard of care.

"Do not count the days; make the days count."

\-   Muhammad Ali

What to Expect

If you or your loved one has been diagnosed with a disease which is considered terminal or life-limiting, there may come a time when your physicians suggest hospice care. This is usually because you have received the maximum treatment for the illness, and/or further treatment is not advised.

The patient may have experienced progression of the disease despite treatment or had multiple hospitalizations or ER visits. They may be having any number of troubling symptoms related to the illness, including pain, weight loss, shortness of breath, poor appetite and others. Chances are that the patient and family are experiencing a great deal of anxiety and stress.

Visits to the primary care doctor's office or the hospital are largely focused on curing the condition; the patient and family may have become frustrated and feel that only temporary relief has been provided. Often the patient and family feel that the patient is suffering and needs much more attention.

A hospice evaluation may come about based on a physician's advice, or a patient/family may decide that they wish to explore this option. In any case, a physician order is necessary for a hospice referral to take place. Once an order is written, a hospice representative will come and speak with the patient and family to answer questions regarding hospice and obtain more information about the patient. This meeting may take place wherever the patient is – a hospital, nursing home or other long-term care facility, or in the patient's home.

If a decision is reached to proceed with hospice admission, the patient or representative will be asked to sign papers for admission. Usually a close family member will be designated as the primary caregiver. The primary caregiver will serve as the main point of contact throughout hospice care and will help to make decisions regarding care.

A registered nurse will do an evaluation on the patient and formulate a plan of care with input from at least one other member of the interdisciplinary team. The admitting nurse will evaluate what the patient's immediate needs are concerning pain and symptom control, as well as equipment and supplies. The nurse will also assess whether the patient requires a nursing aide to help provide care.

In addition, evaluations will be completed by the hospice social worker to assess psychosocial needs; and the hospice chaplain or counselor to assess spiritual/emotional needs. These evaluations will consider the needs of the patient as well as the family.

The above proceedings will take place times and places which are most convenient for the patient and family. It is important to be expedient, however, so that the patient may begin receiving comfort care as soon as possible. Medications, equipment, supplies and the hospice team will be available to the patient as soon as he or she is admitted to hospice.

At a minimum, the nurse is required to visit and assess the hospice patient at least every 14 days. In most cases your hospice nurse will visit the day following admission and at least once weekly to reassess patient condition and needs. In addition, you will receive regular visits from the other members of the hospice team as mentioned. The purpose of these visits is to implement a thoughtfully designed plan of care – tailored to meet the needs of the patient and the family. This plan of care is discussed and updated regularly by the interdisciplinary team, with input from the patient and family.

Hospice services are available to the patient 24 hours a day, seven days a week.

"Hospice is not the fast track to the end of the race…it's simply choosing a smoother ride for the journey."

- Author unknown

Hospice Myths and Reality

Conversations about death and dying really are few and far between – especially considering this is a topic which is relevant to us all. Conversations about hospice are perhaps even more scarce – even among medical professionals.

As a result, there are bound to be misconceptions. Perhaps you have heard some of these yourself. A common myth is that a hospice patient must use a hospice that the doctor or facility refers them to, in reality, a patient has the right to freedom of choice and self-determination to select whichever hospice they deem appropriate for their care. This chapter will discuss more common myths regarding hospice, and the truth of the matter.

I must sign a DNR in order to receive hospice services. A patient is not required to have a DNR (Do Not Resuscitate) in order to receive hospice services. A DNR is a medical order written by a physician prior to a medical crisis, so that caregivers and family are aware that the patient does not desire heroic measures if their heart stops beating, or if they stop breathing.

Please keep in mind that knowing a patient's wishes before they decline to a point where they can no longer communicate can afford you and your family a great deal of comfort and stress relief. Your hospice representative will discuss with you something called an Advance Directive. You may already have an advance directive, such as a living will. An advance directive makes a patient's wishes known concerning treatment in the event of their decline. Your hospice representative will assist you in making an informed choice concerning an advance directive.

Hospice is only for cancer patients. In reality, hospice is for any patient facing any number of medical conditions which could result in death over the next six months. In choosing hospice, these patients choose to forego aggressive treatment for that condition. Many times, these conditions are described as "end-stage," and may affect major organs including the heart, lungs, kidneys, liver or brain. The doctor and a hospice professional will determine if a patient's condition meets criteria for hospice care.

Hospice means that the patient will die soon. In reality, hospice simply provides care for people with limited life expectancy. The general guideline is that the patient may die within about six months if the disease follows its natural course. It does not mean that the patient will die or must die within six months. Some hospice patients pass away much sooner than six months – others pass away after a much longer time. Still others may even be discharged from hospice if their condition is no longer considered terminal.

Hospice means giving up faith and hope. Many times, when patients and their families are faced with a terminal illness, they focus on the impending death – rather than making the most of the life that remains. Hospice does not mean you or your loved one have abandoned faith or given up hope. It is a quality choice to reclaim the spirit of life.

Simply put, hospice provides everything a patient needs to live his or her best life, in an environment that is preferred for patient and family. This means medications, supplies, equipment and staff on call 24 hours a day. Hospice is also is a rich source of physical, emotional and spiritual comfort for both patient and family.

Although thoughts of illness and death can lead to sadness, anger and emotional pain, it can also lead to opportunities for closeness with loved ones; reflection on life issues you would not otherwise have experienced; and times of laughter, reminiscence and happiness.

Once a patient chooses hospice, he or she can no longer see their primary physician or seek treatment at the hospital. In reality, the hospice patient can choose to see his or her primary care physician (PCP) – or seek care at a hospital – at any time. Some PCP's choose to turn over complete care of the patient to the hospice medical director. Others continue to care for the patient in partnership with the hospice team. In either case, hospice places much value on the patient-physician relationship and continues to work closely with the patient's PCP throughout the course of care.

In addition, a patient may seek care at a hospital for any condition not related to the hospice diagnosis. For example, if a patient is admitted to hospice for terminal lung cancer and suffers a broken bone, he may be treated in the hospital for the broken bone, without hospice care being affected.

Hospice patients become addicted to morphine. In reality, hospice patients with limited life expectancy do not have enough time for legitimate concern over addiction to pain medications. Greater concern should be devoted to using the most effective means of comfort for the patient, while allowing for the best quality of life overall. Hospice physicians and nurses are experts at pain/symptom control. They work closely together and with pharmacists to continually develop and use new protocols for keeping patients as comfortable, alert and functional as possible. Morphine is only one of the medications used to accomplish this. The hospice medical professionals discuss patient care on an ongoing basis. They know which medications and combinations of medications provide the best results for each patient.

Hospice stops feeding patients and they become dehydrated and starve to death. In reality, hospice encourages patients to eat and drink only what they want. Although difficult for families to comprehend and accept, it is natural for some patients to not feel hunger or thirst; it is part of how the body shuts down. This topic is further discussed in Chapter 5.

Patients can only receive hospice care for a limited amount of time. In reality, patients can continue to receive hospice services as long as medically necessary, while the disease takes its natural course. This care is paid for by Medicare or most private insurance.

Patients may also be discharged and re-admitted to hospice as needed. You should be aware, however, that this may cause some forfeiture of benefits. Your hospice representative will provide more information on this as needed.

"As the body becomes weaker, so the spirit becomes stronger."

\-   Cicely Saunders

Stages of Decline and Death

You are likely reading this book because you are experiencing a loved one being terminally ill and either contemplating hospice or receiving hospice services now. You have been advised by doctors that the condition or disease state of your loved one is irreversible and, if the disease follows its natural course, it will end in death.

Hospice sees to it that each patient has what is termed a "good death." This may sound disturbing or like an oxymoron. However, many believe that death can be thought of as the ultimate healing – as sickness, pain and suffering come to an end when death occurs.

The way that each person lives his or her life is completely unique. Personality, temperament, career, family life and personal or religious beliefs – these are just a few of the things that make your loved one unique. It is likely also that the journey towards transition will also have its unique aspects.

Stories have been told about and by those who have had near-death experiences. People have even said they believe their loved ones have communicated with them after they have died. But I am confident that no reliable firsthand accounts exist of what death and dying are truly like. However, people who work with hospice patients and their families are acquainted with end-of-life issues and with the dying process. There are many things which have shown themselves to be common to patients approaching death. Understanding these will help you manage with less fear and confusion as your loved one declines.

Following are some general guidelines of what you may see in the weeks, days and hours leading up to your loved one's passing. Please remember that these guidelines are indeed general, and the length of time between hospice admission and death varies widely from patient to patient.

Information here is based on medical and scientific principles, as well as commonly reported experiences of professional hospice caregivers. As your loved one declines, you may observe none, some or all of the events and symptoms discussed in this section.

Do not hesitate to consult a member of your hospice team if you ever feel confused, anxious or have other concerns about what you observe in your loved one.

One to three months before death - Your loved one may seem detached from everyday life. He may not be interested in things he previously found pleasure in. There will be a need to talk less and sleep more. They may even have a faraway look in their eyes, and at times may not seem to be listening when you talk to them. This is the beginning of letting go of life to prepare for death.

Physical changes tend to occur or worsen during this time as well. Weight loss, decreased appetite, and generalized weakness are to be expected. Depending on disease process, other symptoms including pain, shortness of breath or swelling may occur or worsen. The medication used to relieve these symptoms and provide comfort could contribute to the patient sleeping more.

One to two weeks before death - Intake of food and fluids will further decrease and may stop entirely. As the body begins to shut down, food and nutrients become unnecessary. In fact, forcing food and fluids on a patient at this stage burdens the body and can even result in aspiration of food into the lungs, causing airway compromise and/or pneumonia. In a normal person, digestion and metabolism are ongoing processes which we take for granted. In a dying patient these processes have slowed to the point that food will most likely cause vomiting, constipation or both.

Your loved one may speak only a few words each day or may not speak at all. Generalized weakness increases and they often become bedbound. This weakness can lead to bowel and bladder incontinence. But because of less intake of food and fluids, there will be less output of stool and urine. Urine becomes concentrated and dark in color.

Visual and/or auditory hallucinations often occur, particularly as the central nervous system begins to be affected. Sometimes a patient may confuse a particular sound with the sound of a human voice. It is also common for the dying to see visions of other loved ones who have passed on. At times they may seem focused on "another world," and may interact with people or things that cannot be seen by others. Although this may be upsetting for you and others, in hospice this is considered normal.

One to seven days before death – Blood pressure usually decreases and at times the pulse will be irregular. Usually there is an increase in congestion and breathing becomes noisy and/or labored. You may hear gurgling sounds as the patient breaths, due to congestion and the patient being too weak to cough up secretions.

Restlessness and agitation are also common symptoms. This may be caused by decreased oxygen delivery to the brain, metabolic changes, dehydration and pain medications. There are other medications which may be given to promote rest. Be aware, though, that your loved one may exhibit restlessness because he or she might have some unfinished business. Issues may be lingering in the mind or heart, and they may need to achieve a sense of security and completion.

It is also important for you to know that many times a person will show signs of recovery before death takes place. They may suddenly become coherent, even having conversations with others. The appetite may seem to reappear. We call this "rallying," and it does not last long – usually a day or less. When the rallying period is over the final decline usually occurs.

Hours before death - The patient is usually unresponsive; eyes may be open or closed. It may appear as if the patient is staring into space, not really focusing on anything. Breathing patterns will be irregular. There may be periods between breaths, up to 30 seconds or more. This can last from a few minutes to hours.

With blood pressure and pulse rate fluctuating and/or decreasing, blood moves away from the extremities and inward, towards the vital organs. The hands and feet may be cool while the abdomen may be warm. Skin will be pale, but you may see blotchiness or purplish/bluish discoloration on the legs, arms or underside of the patient's body. This is called mottling.

It is very important that you remember that, although your loved one may seem unresponsive, they do have awareness and can hear you speaking to them. We are unaware of studies or scientific proof, but it is widely accepted in the medical community that hearing is the last sense to leave a dying person. Therefore, it is extremely important to speak comforting, loving words to the dying. It is equally important to refrain from speaking anything potentially upsetting to them.

When the dying process is complete, breathing will cease, and the heart will stop. There will be no response to stimulation. The jaw will relax, and the mouth may fall open. There may also be a release of bowel/bladder contents.

Ideally, a member of your hospice team will be present at the time of death. The nurse or medical director will check for pulse and respirations and will confirm that your loved one has passed on. Remember that this is not an emergency so calling 911 is not necessary. Your hospice team member will notify the coroner first. There is no rush to call the funeral home right away.

You may wish to spend some quiet reflective time with your loved one's body. Take time to process what has happened and say your final goodbye. You may choose to bathe and dress your loved one. This should be done within the first hour before the body begins to stiffen. If present, generally your hospice nurse or aide can help if you wish. When the final goodbyes and preparations to the body have been made, the funeral home is notified, and the body removed.

"To make a difference in someone's life you don't have to be brilliant, rich, beautiful, or perfect. You just have to care."

-   Mandy Hale

Comfort You Can Provide

You have hired a very specialized team of trained professionals to care for your loved one in their final days and moments on earth. However, the hospice team recognizes and respects the powerful bonds of relationship, faith and family.

Approaching death may be unfamiliar and frightening to you and your family, but do not underestimate your own ability to give comfort and care to this person you love so dearly. There are many things you can do to make your loved one's passage more dignified and comfortable. Some of them are so simple that you may not have thought of them. The reality is that even the smallest word or action counts!

Your interventions should always be guided by your hospice nurse. Keeping this in mind, consider the following:

- Provide a comforting atmosphere – Try to keep the room and the patient at a comfortable temperature. Sometimes our instinct tells us to cover our loved one with a blanket – but keep in mind that this could be making them feel too warm. Terminal patients may often run fever. If you are wondering, you can check temperature by placing a thermometer in the armpit, keeping in mind that a normal temperature by this method is about a degree lower than the normal oral temperature.

- Provide moisture – Since your loved one may not be eating or drinking, the skin and mucus membranes will be drier than usual. If they are on oxygen, it should be humidified (consult your nurse if need be). Apply creams and lotions to the skin after bathing and as needed. Swabbing the mouth with wet sponges may also be comforting. Apply a non-petroleum moisturizer to the lips.

- Provide soothing sounds – Most likely, you do not enjoy loud or sudden noises when you are ill. Neither will your loved one on hospice. If you choose to play music, audible books or other materials, play them softly. Try not to allow loud or disrupting noises or conversations in your loved one's space. Use your discretion with this; we all know that when family and friends gather, laughter and fellowship can sometimes be a bit loud, but still enjoyable!

- Provide comfortable positioning – Keeping the head of the bed at about a 30-degree angle will help the lungs to expand more easily; it will also decrease the risk of saliva and fluids flowing backwards into the throat or esophagus and causing coughing or choking. Use pillows to position and elevate body parts and provide softness. If lying on his or her side, your loved one may like a pillow between the knees, nestled at the back and/or in the arms.

- Provide quiet presence – Your presence is profound! Simply sitting or standing near your loved one has an effect on them. Whether you speak and/or touch them – or choose not to, the fact that you are there matters. Studies have shown that the mere presence of others has a positive effect on humans.

The bottom line is, always consult your hospice team regarding your loved one's care. But there is no need to feel intimidated. Using good common sense is key in most things, and this experience is no exception.

"Death is a challenge. It tells us not to waste time…It tells us to tell each other right now that we love each other."

- Leo Buscaglia

Saying Goodbye

It is most certainly an understatement to say that saying goodbye to your loved one is difficult. Educating yourself on the process and preparing for the moment are important, but even with preparation and knowledge, witnessing the death of a loved one is an extremely profound experience. It can be difficult and heartbreaking to say the least.

Saying goodbye is an important, personal matter, and the way in which you choose to do it is very individualized. We encourage you to take some time and give the process some thought beforehand. There are some things to keep in mind which may prove helpful to you and your loved ones.

It is good to take advantage of opportunities to say goodbye when the person is awake and communicative. Should your loved one be in a coma or unable to communicate, always assume that they can hear and understand you. Studies have shown that unconscious patients can hear and understand spoken words; they also feel and respond to physical touch. My own wife, who was an ICU nurse for many years, has told me numerous stories of patients who awoke from unconscious states and accurately described things that were said around them while they were unconscious. Therefore, never speak about the dying person as if they were not present.

As stated, the way you choose to say goodbye is a personal decision. Some people are comfortable lying in bed next to their loved one as they say their goodbyes. Others simply want to hold hands. If music or prayer is used to assist the dying, ensure that it is familiar and comforting. Sometimes a gentle whisper in their ear saying, "It's ok to go now. We are going to be ok."

Those who are closest to the dying person may choose to be absent. There are times when a dying person will wait to die until loved ones have left the room. If you feel this is the case with your loved one, simply saying, "I'm going to leave the room for a while. I love you" is all that is needed.

It is also helpful to note that people who are dying frequently want "permission" to pass on from those they love. Often, they want to be assured of five basic things:

- Things they were once responsible for will be taken care of.
- Their survivors will be alright without them.
- All is forgiven.
- Their life had meaning.
- They will be remembered.

Whatever manner you believe is most appropriate in which to say goodbye to your loved one, is the best way. The goodbye is important, to give both you and your beloved a sense of closure. But try not to feel undue stress or anxiety over it. It can be very helpful to discuss this with your hospice chaplain and/or social worker, as they are specially trained in the spiritual and psychosocial aspects of your experience.

"There is a voice that doesn't use words. Listen."

\-   Rumi

Hear My Voice

Years ago, I was at the bedside of one of my closest friends and colleagues, Chaplain Stephen Murphy, as he lay dying of cancer. The moments were surreal, because Chaplain Murphy and I had been at countless bedsides together, ministering to the dying and their families. We had discussed the care of countless patients during countless interdisciplinary meetings, and Chaplain Murphy had spoken countless prayers to begin our work weeks, to close meetings…to dispel fear and bring comfort to souls as they approached the threshold of death.

He was relatively young, had a beautiful wife and two young adult children. Before cancer entered his life, he was a robust, hard-working hospice chaplain and pastor of his own church.

And now, as Chaplain Murphy lay in his own bed preparing to cross that very threshold himself, he was speaking to me. I could tell that he was expressing to me his love and concern for his family, his awareness that he would soon pass away.

As he spoke to me, it was difficult to understand him over the continuous rush of oxygen through the mask. He seemed to know this, because he beckoned me to come closer. As I leaned in, I heard Chaplain Murphy's instruction: "Just hear my voice."

Just Hear My Voice.

In many ways, sickness and death have been a place of equality since the beginning of time – for the dying and for his or her loved ones. Just as disease and death don't discriminate, neither do heartache and grief. As you walk through your own difficult trial, listen for the voice of your loved one. Be mindful of all the ways they communicate their needs. Aside from life itself, this is the most important journey they will ever make. At times their needs may be quite different from what we may think or desire for them.

As you help in managing end-of-life care for your beloved, you will make decisions, react to events and face many circumstances. Remember that the comfort and dignity of your loved one comes before all else. Be guided by conversations you have had with them, as well as what you know about their particular personality and desires. During their time on hospice, you will also become acquainted with non-verbal cues which indicate certain needs. Be guided by all this, as well as your hospice team and this book, to determine and fulfill those needs.

You are in a position of exquisite difficulty and privilege. You are helping to ensure that your loved one transitions from this life with the greatest degree of comfort and dignity possible. There is no doubt that the comfort you provide now will return to serve you after your loved one has passed on.

"Grief is not a disorder, a disease or a sign of weakness. It is an emotional, physical and spiritual necessity, the price you pay for love..."

-   Earl Grollman

Acknowledgements

I thank my wife of 32 years, Linda Cox, mother to my sons, closest friend, and a gifted nurse practitioner in hospice and overall.

Chaplain Mark Eakin, my forever friend whom St. Mark Hospice is named after. How I wish you were here to use your gifts in the business.

David Nelson, MD, who over the years has tirelessly provided his medical/clinical expertise, as well as his commitment to hospice care.

Hospice chaplain Stephen Murphy – taken too soon and in the midst of service to his family, to hospice and to the ministry.

My beloved mother Mary Cox, my dearest mentor in all things pertaining to life;

My godparents Dr. Dennis and Clara Brooks, whose steadfast love and guidance have been more valuable to me than silver and gold;

My late father-in-law George Verrett, possibly my most endearing hospice patient of all – yet dear to me for so many more reasons.

Jessie Williams, your name is forever etched in my heart and mind, because you were my very first hospice patient.

And my sons Jerome II, Ryan, George and Adam – my right-hand men in the business of life.

Notes

Notes

Notes

Made in the USA
Columbia, SC
05 February 2020